BEN

DYSLEXIA
Pocketbook

By Julie Bennett

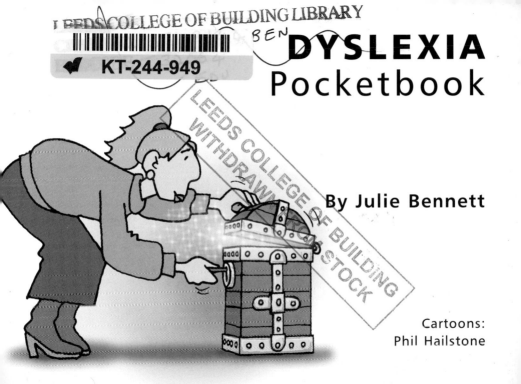

Cartoons:
Phil Hailstone

Published by:

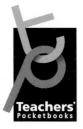

Teachers' Pocketbooks
Laurel House, Station Approach,
Alresford, Hampshire SO24 9JH, UK
Tel: +44 (0)1962 735573
Fax: +44 (0)1962 733637
E-mail: sales@teacherspocketbooks.co.uk
Website: www.teacherspocketbooks.co.uk

*Teachers' Pocketbooks is an imprint of
Management Pocketbooks Ltd.*

Series Consultant: **Brin Best**.

ISBN 9 781903 776681
ISBN 1 903776 68 6

British Library Cataloguing-in-Publication
Data – A catalogue record for this book is
available from the British Library.

Design, typesetting and graphics by Efex Ltd.
Printed in UK.

Contents

Foreword

When I first began teaching, nearly 20 years ago, it was common to be told there was no such thing as dyslexia, or that it was 'a middle class excuse for failure to learn to read and write'. Although these views are gradually disappearing as more research is done in the field of dyslexia, there is continuing discussion about its:

- Definition
- Terminology
- Causes
- Nature and characteristics

I welcome the recent call for clarity over the definition of dyslexia and look forward to the day when we have a worldwide definition, uniform assessment criteria and equal provision for people with dyslexia. In the meantime, it is worth emphasising:

Dyslexia itself is not a myth, but there are myths about dyslexia.

Foreword

Dyslexia is **NOT**:

✗ Simply a reading issue
✗ An excuse (middle class or other) for a lazy child
✗ A ruse to get preferential treatment
✗ A result of low IQ

The impact of dyslexia is **real**. It affects many millions of children and adults around the world in their acquisition of literacy and numeracy skills and in the way they function in everyday life. Dyslexic learners often say they feel they don't seem to 'fit' into the world. They frequently devise creative and ingenious solutions to overcome their difficulties. Effective teachers nurture this in their learners by enabling them to

- Develop **strategies** to match their differences
- Recognise that they have **strengths** which are valued in society
- Develop a **positive self-image**, despite their learning differences

Foreword

This book is based on the growing understanding of how dyslexia affects children's learning and the **strategies** we can put in place to alleviate their difficulties and maximise their strengths. It's a **practical** guide for non-specialist teachers and teaching assistants. Parents may also find it useful. It will provide you with:

- An outline of what **dyslexia** is
- Information about **learning profiles** of dyslexic students
- Suggested **solutions** and **practical techniques**
- Ways to help you **improve the performance** of your dyslexic students
- An overview of some **different approaches** to dyslexia
- Pointers to further **resources**

The research and debate about dyslexia will continue. Meanwhile, the overriding issue is to keep finding practical ways of assisting dyslexic students to overcome their learning barriers and unlock their potential. This book is designed to build on your strengths as a teacher and give you more resources to help you nurture **independent, resourceful** dyslexic learners.

Introduction

ABLE to influence

As teachers we know that we are in a position of influence.
Our **A**ttitudes **B**eliefs and **L**anguage have an **E**ffect on those we are working with.

Good teachers recognise that if they consider a dyslexic student to be 'lazy' or 'stupid', their attitudes, beliefs and language will negatively affect their interaction with that student.

On the other hand, the attitudes, beliefs and language of teachers who consider their students to be full of potential, each having something valuable to offer, will positively affect their interaction with them. This principle contributes to my approach to dyslexia in the classroom.

Throughout the book I use the term **'learning difference'** rather than learning disability. This highlights that dyslexic learners have a different way of processing information.

Outcomes

Teachers often tell me that one of the biggest challenges they face in the classroom is the fact that dyslexic students are so dependent on the teacher. Taking an holistic approach to their needs allows them to develop their independence.

Approaching dyslexia effectively nurtures:

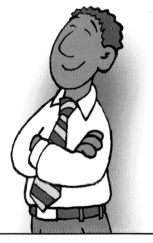

- Resourcefulness and strategic learning
- Resilience and confidence
- Responsibility and independence
- Respect for self and others
- Reflection and reasoning

Much of the advice in this book for teaching dyslexic learners will encompass the wider needs of your class, as some of the characteristics of dyslexic students are likely to be found in other students too. You'll find there are tools, techniques and methods here for working with individuals, small groups and whole classes.

Roots and wings

There is an old saying:

'The two most valuable things we can give our children are:

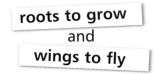

roots to grow
and
wings to fly

This is a useful image on which to build a model for approaching dyslexia in the classroom.

The **roots** are the areas we need to focus on as teachers, in order to provide strong foundations of effective learning for dyslexics.

The **wings** illustrate the outcomes of effective learning, in other words the qualities that will be nurtured in our dyslexic learners.

Roots and wings

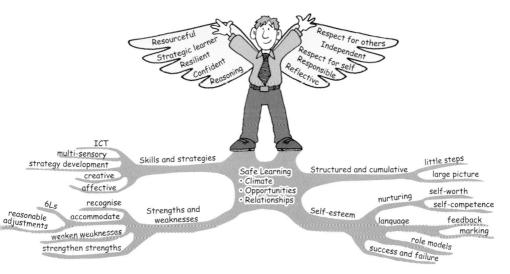

Resourceful
Strategic learner
Resilient
Confident
Reasoning

Respect for others
Independent
Respect for self
Responsible
Reflective

ICT
multi-sensory
strategy development
creative
affective

Skills and strategies

Safe Learning
• Climate
• Opportunities
• Relationships

Structured and cumulative

little steps
large picture

6Ls
reasonable adjustments
recognise
accommodate
weaken weaknesses
strengthen strengths

Strengths and weaknesses

Self-esteem

nurturing

self-worth
self-competence

lanquage

feedback
marking

role models
success and failure

Safe learning

In the diagram on page 11, the trunk or main part of the roots represents the need for 'safe learning'.

Imagine starting your lesson and discovering that Darren has let his venomous pet snake loose. Your **sense of safety** is **threatened** and you feel insecure; you lose your focus and concentration.

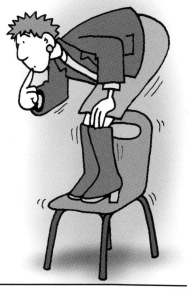

A similar event occurs for dyslexics: in the classroom they fear **failure** and **humiliation**. This has a dramatic effect on their learning. What happens is that fear triggers a **fight or flight** response where the learner experiences stress and learning becomes more difficult.

Climate, relationships, opportunities

There are three interconnected elements of safe learning which teachers can provide:

1. Climate
2. Relationships
3. Opportunities

Climate

We can provide a positive climate where it is safe to take learning risks and possibly make mistakes. Failure is seen as part of the learning process rather than the end-product of an unsuccessful learning experience.

Relationships

We can nurture safe relationships between ourselves and students and among students in the class. These relationships are founded on respect for individuals and belief in their potential. The higher the teacher's emotional intelligence and self-esteem, the greater the development of student self-esteem.

Climate, relationships, opportunities

Opportunities

We can create opportunities which take into consideration the needs of dyslexic learners. These learning opportunities will aim to 'strengthen dyslexic strengths and weaken dyslexic weaknesses'. They will make reasonable adjustments for dyslexic difficulties and provide appropriately matched strategies to develop skills. They will be structured and cumulative, building on previous learning and at the same time giving an overview of the whole learning context.

If we develop these three aspects of 'safe' learning, our students will feel that it's okay to take learning risks and begin to unlock their potential.

What is
Dyslexia?

Difficulty with words

The word 'dyslexia' has a Greek origin.

- 'Dys' means 'difficulty'
- 'Lexia' comes from the root 'lexis' which means 'words or language'

At its simplest, dyslexia means 'difficulty with words or language'. It is important, though, to take the term 'language' to have a broad all-embracing meaning. Many people think that dyslexia is just a reading or spelling problem, but in fact it's often a difficulty with language in the forms of:

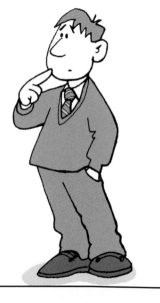

- Spelling
- Writing
- Speaking
- Reading
- Processing
- Organisation
- Memory

Definition

Worldwide, there is no single, commonly accepted definition of dyslexia.
This is the one I have found most useful:

'Dyslexia is best described as a combination of abilities and difficulties which affect the learning process in one or more of reading, spelling and writing. Accompanying weaknesses may be identified in areas of speed of processing, short-term memory, sequencing and organisation, auditory and or visual perception, spoken language and motor skills. It is particularly related to mastering and using written language, which may include alphabetic, numeric and musical notation. Some children have outstanding creative skills, others have strong oral skills. Some have no outstanding talents. All have strengths. Dyslexia can occur despite intellectual ability and conventional teaching. It is independent of socio, economic or language background.'

Dr. Lindsay Peer, CBE
International Dyslexia Consultant, formerly BDA Education Director and Deputy Chief Executive of the British Dyslexia Association (BDA) email: lindsaypeer@hotmail.com

Terminology

The terms you are most likely to come across as teachers are:

- **Dyslexia** and
- **Specific Learning Difficulty** (SpLD)

You may well also come across the phrase **developmental dyslexia**, perhaps in psychologist reports.

You will possibly have heard of people who have had a head injury or a stroke and then become dyslexic. This is another type of dyslexia called **acquired dyslexia**. The dyslexia is *acquired* through brain injury or illness.

In this book I use the term '**dyslexia**' (referring to developmental dyslexia) as one of many **specific learning difficulties** such as dyspraxia, dyscalculia, ADHD etc.

A collection of differences

It is helpful to build up a picture of the condition and how it affects learners. Dyslexia is:

- A learning 'difference'
- A pattern of weaknesses and strengths
- A processing difference

It can be seen as a syndrome – a collection of **differences** in learning, including **weaknesses** and **strengths**.

Not all dyslexics experience the same weaknesses or strengths.

Solving the puzzle

For a better understanding it is helpful to take a closer look at the four components of the dyslexic profile.

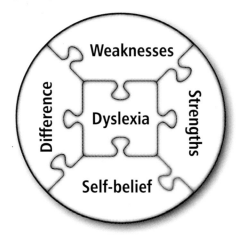

Difference

Dyslexia is a learning difference. There are many suppositions about its causes, not all of which are founded in science. However, there is scientific understanding about dyslexia and this page provides you with the key words to use if you would like to find out more about the research.

Scientific research has shown that compared with patterns noticed in 'non dyslexics', people with 'dyslexia' have differences in:

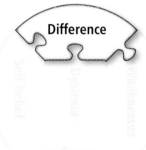

- **Patterns of brain activity**
- **Genetic make up**. Scientists have identified some of the **chromosomes** which are probably linked to dyslexia
- The way the **cerebellum** and the **corpus callosum** function
- **The development of large neurons** (magnocells)

- **Neural connections**
- **Processing styles**
- **Brain reaction to phonological and visual information**

Marked difference

Using the model of dyslexia as *a different way of processing, thinking and learning* helps to establish dyslexia as a 'difference' rather than a 'disability' and opens up the possibility for us to consider strengths as well as weaknesses.

There is another key 'difference', this time related to the assessment and identification of dyslexia:

the marked difference between a child's potential and his/her written work.

The effects of these differences will be highlighted when considering the other three components of the dyslexic puzzle: **weaknesses**, **strengths** and **self-belief**.

Weaknesses

This is the area that you are most likely to notice first
when you have dyslexic students in your class.
Weaknesses show up in the following areas:

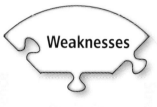

- Reading
- Writing
- Spelling
- Numeracy
- Speaking and listening
- Learning to read musical notation
- Organisation
- Time management

Weaknesses and difficulties

The pattern of weaknesses may include some of the following:

- **Speed of processing** – information is processed more slowly
- **Short-term memory** – difficulty retaining information in short-term or working memory, eg the student forgets what you have just asked him/her to do, especially if given more than one instruction at a time
- **Sequencing** – difficulty putting things in order, such as days of week, numbers, and letters. This may be referred to as visual or auditory sequencing memory. It is related to difficulties in **automaticity**, ie automatically recalling sequences
- **Auditory perception and processing** – difficulty in perceiving, discriminating and processing what is heard: sounds, syllables, words, sentences (phonological difficulties); muddled pronunciation, eg 'par cark' for 'car park', 'pacific' for 'specific' and confusion of similar sounds, such as 'our' and 'are'

Weaknesses and difficulties

- **Visual perception and processing** – difficulty in perceiving, discriminating and processing what is seen: letter shapes, words, sentences (graphemic difficulties); muddling similar-looking words such as 'horse' and 'house'
- **Visual disturbance** – eg words seem wobbly, may have difficulties tracking text from one line to the next
- **Laterality difficulties** – may have difficulties consistently remembering which is left and right hand; reversing of symbols 'b/d' or writing 'god' as 'dog'; may experience some directional difficulties, losing way around school or town, for instance
- **Organisation** – difficulty organising materials, self and thoughts; particular difficulties with organising thoughts to get them down on paper
- **Spoken language** – difficulty getting thoughts out as words. May be noticed in lack of fluent expression or apparently disorganised or disjointed conversation

Weaknesses and difficulties

- **Word naming** – difficulty in finding the name for something known, eg *'I need that 'thingamy' over there'*
- **Decoding written language** – either a phonemic or graphemic difficulty. A **phonemic** difficulty (sometimes known as phonological processing deficit) is related to the sounds of letters and words. A **graphemic** difficulty is related to the way letters and words look and are processed
- **Motor co-ordination** – may have poor co-ordination with
  - Gross motor movements, eg catching a ball
  - Fine motor movements, eg using scissors
  - Grapho motor movements, eg handwriting

Some dyslexic learners may also have **dyspraxia** (also known as developmental co-ordination disorder or DCD) which is a difficulty with the organisation of movement.

Fortunately, weaknesses do not make up the whole picture. There are more parts of the dyslexia puzzle to consider.

Strengths

The work of various researchers points to the possibility of dyslexics having enhanced functioning in areas such as **visual/spatial skills** and **creativity**. This may explain why dyslexic learners often display talent in areas such as arts, photography, mechanics, sport, engineering, etc.

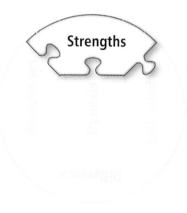

These **patterns of strengths** may have developed because an individual has come across difficulties and developed new, creative ways of doing things, or it may be that their creative skills are an inbuilt, innate part of the dyslexic profile.

Either way, the importance is that strengths do exist. You may well be able to identify these skills in the people you know to be dyslexic.

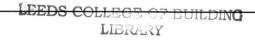

Patterns of strengths

Students with dyslexia may have enhanced function and ability in

- Grasping an overview
- Visualisation
- Art
- Articulation
- Visual-spatial skills
- Imagination
- Creativity
- Multi-tasking
- Making unexpected links, associations or applications
- Free thinking
- People skills
- Design

- 3D thinking
- Visionary thinking
- Problem solving
- Innovation
- Intuition

Increased abilities

Focusing on these aspects of the dyslexic profile makes it easier to know how to help dyslexic learners reach their potential.

These increased abilities can be employed to improve learning opportunities. Many of the dyslexics in our classes are likely to learn well in ways which involve

- Creativity
- Team work
- Lateral thinking
- Pictures
- Themes

- Implicit learning
- Solving problems
- Sub-conscious learning
- 3-dimensional thinking
- Intuition

Knowing this helps us to adjust the methods we use to activate learning and the way we deliver information.

Nurturing success

When working with dyslexic learners, aim to:

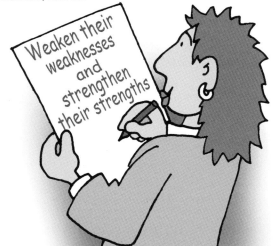

Weaken their weaknesses and strengthen their strengths

This book explores ways of doing this by focusing on their strengths as well as their weaknesses.

Most importantly, we can show our learners that people with dyslexia can be successful......

Success stories

There are a good number of successful people in the public eye who are reported to be dyslexic:

Paul Smith (fashion designer)
Sir Jackie Stewart (racing driver)
Benjamin Zephaniah (poet)
Duncan Goodhew (swimmer)
Sir Steve Redgrave (rower)

Eddie Izzard (comedian)
Zoë Wanamaker (actress)
Richard Branson (entrepreneur)
Susan Hampshire (actress)
Lee Ryan (singer)

Some historical figures thought to have been dyslexic include:

Albert Einstein (physicist)
Henry Ford (inventor)
Leonardo Da Vinci (artist and inventor)
Thomas Alva Edison (scientist and inventor)
Winston Churchill (politician)

Negative self-belief

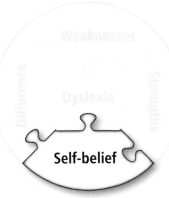

Despite the fact that dyslexics have strengths, they often struggle to believe positive things about themselves as learners. This leads to **low self-esteem and self-confidence.**

You can recognise low levels of self-belief in the classroom by noticing a pattern of difficulties accompanied by persistent:

- Lack of confidence
- Reluctance to answer questions
- Poor motivation
- Disruptive behaviour
- Unfavourable comparison of themselves with their peers
- Shyness or being the class joker

Self-belief and learning

We know that:

- Negative self-belief **adversely affects learning**
- Dyslexic difficulties seem to **get worse** when the dyslexic learner is under **stress**
- Negative self-belief places **limits on performance**

Dyslexics often feel emotions related to their negative self-belief and self-concept as learners. They may question their worth and may experience:

- A sense of **failure** in the classroom
- A sense of **isolation**
- A sense of being **overwhelmed**
- **Lack of motivation**

If dyslexia is addressed early in a child's school life, they may escape many of these negative feelings. However, it's never too late. The next chapter shows how you can work with learners of all ages to build self-esteem and boost confidence.

Setting them up for success

With this pattern of:

Difference + Weaknesses + Strengths + Self-belief

there is an opportunity for dyslexics to **succeed or fail** as learners. Much of our education system is geared towards literacy and numeracy and many of the weaknesses of dyslexics are related to literacy and numeracy. Immediately, there is potential for repeated failure.

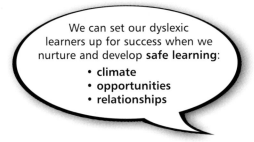

We can set our dyslexic learners up for success when we nurture and develop **safe learning**:
- **climate**
- **opportunities**
- **relationships**

Dyslexia and Self-esteem

Self-esteem is not fixed

Experience of working with dyslexic learners, anecdotal evidence and research tell us that dyslexics are susceptible to

- Low self-esteem
- Distorted self-concepts
- Low confidence

However, not all dyslexics have low self-esteem and, importantly, self-esteem is not fixed. Our learners are capable of changing and enhancing their estimation of themselves and raising their levels of confidence.

Self-worth and self-competence

Self-esteem involves two aspects: **self-worth** and **self-competence**.

People with **low self-esteem** believe that they are:

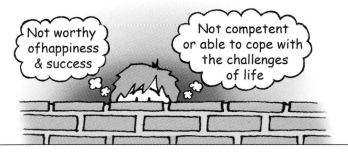

Not worthy of happiness & success

Not competent or able to cope with the challenges of life

Low self-esteem causes problems for learners. Their confidence diminishes and this becomes a learning barrier.

(Based on Nathaniel Branden's work *Six Pillars of Self-Esteem*, Bantam,1994)

Patterns of thinking

Some dyslexic learners develop **patterns of thinking** that contribute to establishing low self-esteem.

These learners will be **internalising** the reasons for certain things that happen in the world as **their fault**. They subsequently **blame** themselves, feel **shame** and draw conclusions about themselves which diminish their self-worth and competence.

They will be **filtering** their interactions with others, looking for **negative feedback** and focusing on that. They are going to be experts **at discounting the positives** you feed back to them.

Context

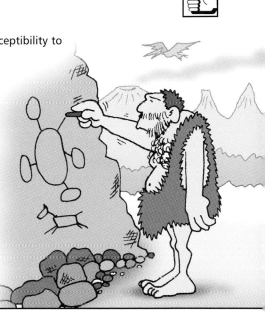

Another contributing factor to dyslexics' susceptibility to developing low self-esteem is **context**.

Imagine, for a moment, the dyslexic in a pre-literate society – one where reading and writing played little part. The difficulties faced by dyslexic learners may well have gone unnoticed. We may instead have noticed their skills and talents in creative, kinaesthetic activities.

A repeated cycle

Dyslexics are working in an environment which, for a large proportion of time, focuses on the very thing they are weakest at. Their weaknesses are often highlighted by the ways they are taught (predominantly auditory/visual) and expected to give evidence of their learning (predominantly auditory/visual).

The experience of dyslexics within the education system is often one of **failure**. Failure affects dyslexics negatively (and any one else who has learning differences) because of the **meaning** they make from their experiences within the context.

For the dyslexic learner failure is often a daily **repeated cycle**. The failure cycle has most impact when there is an underlying belief such as: "failure is bad and only bad people fail".

The failure cycle

Enabling our dyslexic learners to develop enhanced self-esteem means:

* Setting them up for success rather than failure
* Reframing the meaning of failure

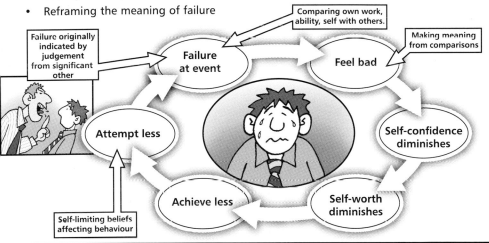

Failure originally indicated by judgement from significant other

Comparing own work, ability, self with others.

Failure at event

Making meaning from comparisons

Feel bad

Self-confidence diminishes

Attempt less

Self-worth diminishes

Achieve less

Self-limiting beliefs affecting behaviour

Reframing failure

Failure in itself is not a 'bad' thing. What has an unhelpful effect on learners is the **negative meaning** they often give to failure, the view of it as the end result of a failed learning experience. I believe we should see failure as an **integral and natural part of the learning process**.

Take learning to ride a bike, for example. If I fall off my bike as I approach a brick wall too fast, I can learn that I am performing an inappropriate set of behaviours which doesn't achieve my goal of staying on the bike. I need to be able to see:

- What I am aiming for
- Why I did not achieve it
- What I need to do differently to improve my skills

The failure of 'falling off' acts as the feedback to help me progress. This is so in any learning experience.

The language of feedback

The feedback you give to your learners is vitally important in helping them to learn from failures and raise their self-esteem. Feedback is most effective when you

Are specific
'Gemma, the way you describe the cricket match is extremely effective because you paint a picture of a typical summer's day.'

Relate the feedback to the learning target
'You have achieved all the targets we set: it is legible, on the line, all the letters are joined up and all the descenders are parallel.'

Ask questions of the learner
'What do you think Grandma would say about the way you have blended your colours here?'
'How proud do you feel of this?'
'Is there one thing you think you could improve on?'

The language of feedback

Give specific guidelines or tips for improving

✗ *'That's no good! Go and do it again'* – doesn't assist the learner in knowing what they have failed to do or how they can improve.

✓ *'If you re-read your writing for capitals and full stops it will improve the way we can read it.'*

Sandwich the constructive criticism between two pieces of praise
If you give feedback which ends negatively, the dyslexic learner will almost certainly remember the last thing you said and may feel negative about their work:

✗ *'That's an imaginative story but there are lots of spelling mistakes.'*

✓ *'It's very imaginative, there are some spelling mistakes, and you have planned the story very well.'*

Comment on the work not the person

✗ *'You are a bad speller.'*

✓ *'You have made some spelling mistakes.'*

Marking

Similarly, the way you mark work has a big impact on how your learners respond to their mistakes.

Consider: are you marking to highlight one area? Or are you aiming to correct every possible aspect of construction, grammar, spelling, and content? How would you feel if you had been faced with a page of your work with every error marked?

Colours
Try marking in two different coloured pens: green for content and blue for spellings.

Tips and Ticks
Try giving ticks for positives and tips written in thought bubbles or drawn in circles.

One by One
Try marking work for one thing at a time: just spelling or just content. See also COPS method (Page 69)

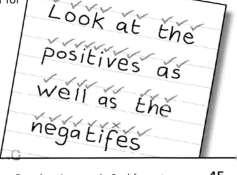

Role models

We are role models for our learners. In the context of failure in learning we can:

- Demonstrate that **failure** is not the most terrible thing in the world
- Demonstrate how to **recover** from failure
- Ensure that children are shown **respect** and not laughed at or ridiculed for failure by peers or teachers
- Allow our learners to hear our **self-talk** related to failure: *'Oh! I spelt that word wrong! Never mind, we all make mistakes! Let's look it up!'*

In doing so we provide our students with a model of:

✓ How to see failure as a positive part of the learning process
✓ How to learn from the failure
✓ How to feel good about themselves as learners

The key to raising self-esteem

It is often said that the most important factor in raising self-esteem is the quality of the relationship a child has with a significant other, eg a teacher, parent, grandparent or carer. As a teacher you are **ABLE** to influence your students' self-worth and self-competence by

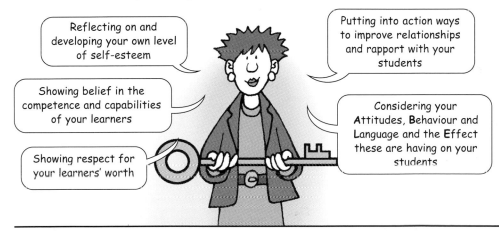

Reflecting on and developing your own level of self-esteem

Putting into action ways to improve relationships and rapport with your students

Showing belief in the competence and capabilities of your learners

Considering your **A**ttitudes, **B**ehaviour and **L**anguage and the **E**ffect these are having on your students

Showing respect for your learners' worth

How do they feel in your classroom?

When asked about what makes a good teacher for dyslexic learners, a 13-year-old replied:

> 'The good teachers make me feel like I'm their friend; the bad teachers make me feel like I'm an **'It'**!'

What sort of relationships do you have with your dyslexic learners?

Introduction

 What is Dyslexia?

 Dyslexia and Self-esteem

 Multi-sensory Learning ◀

 Teaching Tools and Tips

 The 6 Ls

 Current Approaches

 Further Resources

Multi-sensory Learning

Why multi-sensory learning?

When you teach to students' weaknesses, using methods they find difficult, they will struggle. If you apply techniques which use learners' strengths to overcome their weaknesses, you are more likely to end up with students who feel safe in the learning environment and who learn more effectively.

This is why multi-sensory learning is so effective with dyslexic learners. They usually have a particular difficulty in auditory or visual processing (or both). By ensuring the other senses are utilised in teaching and learning you will be enhancing their learning and memory. You will find it also benefits your non-dyslexic learners.

Within the field of dyslexia, multi-sensory teaching was first developed by Gillingham and Stillman in the 1930's. This work became the foundation for multi-sensory teaching and has inspired learning programmes and approaches such as those developed by Hickey and Hornsby. (There is a list of currently available structured multi-sensory literacy programmes on page 120.)

What is multi-sensory learning?

Multi-sensory learning makes use of all the senses: **V**isual (seeing), **A**uditory (hearing), **K**inaesthetic (movement and touch), **O**lfactory (smell) and **G**ustatory (taste): **VAKOG**. The essence of multi-sensory learning is that we provide the best learning opportunities if we teach in a way which involves our learners in as many of the activities below as we can.

Multi-sensory methods are effective for dyslexics because they allow learners to use the methods they are good at while at the same time exercising the methods they are weaker at.

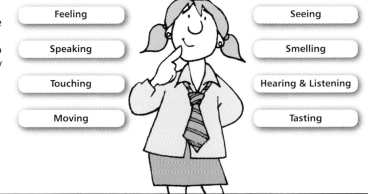

Feeling

Speaking

Touching

Moving

Seeing

Smelling

Hearing & Listening

Tasting

VAK

The different senses we use to take in and process information are sometimes called representational (rep) systems.

Some of our understanding about these comes from the field of NLP (Neuro Linguistic Programming) and the work of Richard Bandler and John Grinder. The NLP theory of rep systems proposes that (unless there is a physical impairment) we use all five senses to take in and process information around us. Although their work was not specific to dyslexia, it is useful to apply their findings to the classroom situation to raise our awareness of learning processes and develop the language we use. This will benefit both dyslexic and non-dyslexic learners.

It is thought that there are three primary channels through which information is taken in: Visual, Auditory and Kinaesthetic (VAK). The language students use reveals clues about which senses they prefer to use as a rep system at a given time.

Find the clues

These clues can help you to modify your teaching so that it is appealing to the preferences and strengths of all learners. The words we use indicate the way we think. Listen for phrases such as those listed in the table below.

Visual	Auditory	Kinaesthetic	Non specific
I can't get the focus of what we're doing.	That's all Greek to me.	I can't put my finger on it.	I don't understand.
I see what you mean.	I hear what you say.	I get the hang of that.	I know what you mean.
Do you think it looks alright?	Does that sound right?	How does that strike you?	How does that seem to you?
I see where you're coming from.	That rings a bell.	I catch your drift.	I understand.

By listening to your students you can pick up an indication of the rep systems they are using. You may find it effective to mirror them. The next page gives some examples of language that appeal to each of the three main learning channels.

Multi-sensory language

The most effective communication uses **a combination of all three rep systems.**

Visual	Auditory	Kinaesthetic	Non specific / all embracing
I want you to focus on what I'm going to show you.	I want you to listen carefully.	I want to put you in touch with this idea.	I want to let you know how to do this.
That's a graphic description!	That's a clear account!	That makes a big impression on the reader!	I get a real sense of excitement from your writing.
Would you illustrate your thinking in an essay?	Would you compose your thoughts on paper now?	Would you help me get a handle on that by putting it down on paper?	Would you explain that in your essay?
That looks like a great idea!	Wow! That sounds like a fantastic idea!	That feels about right to me.	That seems like a great idea!

Using this variety in language can create good rapport between you and your learners. And if you use non-specific language some of the time, you then appeal to all learners. You can affect your learners by the language you use and the type of activities you ask them to do.

Putting it into action

The most successful learning occurs when we use as **many different senses as possible.** For example, a letter shape and its corresponding sound will be best learned by

Seeing and observing the letter shape

Feeling and handling 2D and 3D representation in clay, wood, plastic, sand etc

Hearing own voice or other saying the sound of the letter

Saying or singing the sound of the letter

Moving – making and tracing the letter shape using large and small movements

Smelling the dough/clay etc

Tasting – eating the baked dough shape

Methods like this are effective in strengthening the weaker skills of students with dyslexia. They are techniques that can be transferred to other subjects at all levels.

Multi-sensory teaching

Traditionally, school has been a place where auditory and visual methods of conveying information have been used. A useful way of evaluating lessons with your dyslexic learners in mind is to consider which senses you use in your lessons. Do your learners have a truly multi-sensory experience? Which of these are dominant?

Primary sensory methods of learning:

Visual   - Graphs, pictures, colours, diagrams, mapping, visualisation, film...
Auditory   - Talking, listening, audio recording, music, discussion, explaining...
Kinaesthetic - Movement, activity, handling items, acting, making models, sorting...

Other sensory methods of learning:

Olfactory   - Smelling
Gustatory   - Tasting

Pigeon hole warning!
Using VAK techniques can help to make learning more appropriate for our students but it is not designed to categorise them. It can limit learning if we 'pigeon hole' our learners.

Visual activities

Suggestions for visual learning:

- Diagrams
- Pictures
- Video clips
- Visualisation – *'Can you imagine what that would look like?'*
- Mind Mapping®*
- Doodling on task, drawing or cartoon representation of information or instructions
- Colour – highlighters, different pen colours, highlighter tape, colour coding papers or sections
- Writing or drawing instructions as symbols or key words on to the whiteboard, Post-it® notes or cards

*Mind Map and Mind Mapping are registered trademarks of the Buzan organisation.

Auditory activities

Try getting your students to use some of the following:

- Talking to themselves (internally or on Dictaphone) and to others
- Verbal summaries of key points
- Explanations to another student
- Listening to others
- Sound effects – puppets with funny voices, imagined characters (good for learning spellings)

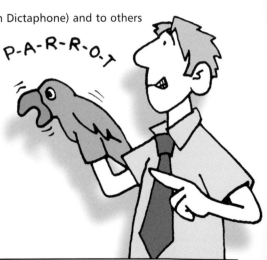

Auditory activities

- Discussion – pairs or groups
- Clips from film, TV or radio
- Rhymes and jingles
- Music, songs, raps
- Voice recording of homework instructions, content, revision...
- Auditory imagination – *'Imagine you can hear... What would it sound like?'*

Auditory activities – music

You can use music to enhance learning:

- Before a learning session
- During a review of material learned (concert review)
- As background music during a particular task
- During a short break in learning
- To introduce themes
- To create a particular learning state – calming, energising, focused

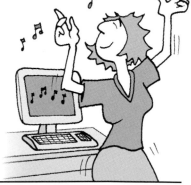

Make sure you pay attention to any students who experience **hearing** or **auditory processing difficulties.** They may find that the background noise is too much for them and you will need to adjust their position, the level of sound etc.

For more information about using music as an aid for all learners:
Mozart effect: www.mozarteffect.com
Sound Health Series: www.advancedbrain.co.uk

Kinaesthetic activities

Try to include some of the following:

- Note-making whilst the learner is hearing information: visual mapping, doodling on task or cartoon representation
- Moving positions, learning in places other than just a desk or table; walking around while learning new information
- Creating short physical breaks, eg stand up, turn around – stretch – then focus
- Writing or drawing key words or pictures on cards, juggling and sorting them
- Hands-on activities, eg human prefixes or suffixes
- Kinaesthetic imagination: *'Imagine how that would feel? How might you act on this?'*
- Role play, experiments, models
- Movement, dance, rhythm

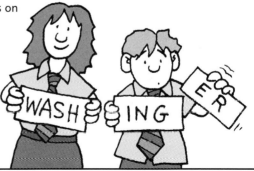

Sit still and listen to me

Learners who have a strong kinaesthetic preference will find it quite difficult to **sit still** and remain **focused**.

Traditionally, we have asked our learners: *'Sit still and look at me when I am talking'*. This may help some students; however in my experience this enables some students to concentrate on looking at my face rather than listening to what I am saying. Research has shown that for some learners, eye contact during 'instruction giving' can be a distraction rather than a help.

You may have noticed that some of your dyslexic students seem to fidget and fiddle a lot. (This also applies to learners with ADHD) You might like to try giving them a small piece of 'Blue Tack' or some small 'stretchy toys' to hold whilst they are listening to you. This seems to help them to focus on what you are saying while keeping their hands engaged in an activity. A good UK supplier of these is www.netfysh.com. This method works well with all ages.

Taste and smell

The following can be used during learning and again to help recall. Your students will associate what they have learned with the smell.

- Lemon or orange cut in half and squeezed into a dish
- Lavender oil sprinkled on a hanky
- Chocolate, bananas, fruity flavoured sweets
- Herbs crushed to enhance smell, eg rosemary, sage, mint
- Orange-scented air spray, room perfumes

For example: a student studies a science module whilst smelling and/or tasting lemon. The student either imagines the smell of lemons when recalling the information learnt or has a small amount of lemon juice placed on the wrist to sniff when recalling the information. This can trigger the memory and assist with recall.

A word of caution: Ensure that students do not react badly (eg asthma sufferers) or are not allergic to particular foods or smells before using this kind of activity.

Taste and smell

Research has suggested that if you encourage your students to

- **Suck peppermints** – it raises alertness by changing brainwaves
- **Drink water** – it hydrates the body and helps concentration
- **Chew gum** – it improves memory

You could try making up 'sensory baskets' to keep in the classroom, eg:

- **Woodland** – cones, leaves, twigs
- **Seaside** – shells, sand, seaweed
- **Grandma's box** – scarf with perfume, pearls, knitting yarn

These baskets can be linked to your subject, starting points for creative writing, or simply sensory stimulation. You could include scented wooden balls, potpourri etc.

Teaching Tools and Tips

Toolkit

In this chapter you will find examples of some of the more **effective tools**, **techniques and tips** to use with dyslexic learners. Many of them use aspects of multi-sensory learning.

The theory behind each technique is relevant to all ages, though you may need to adapt the methods depending on the age group, the subject and your desired outcomes.

The learning tools and techniques in this chapter are for teaching strategies and developing skills that:

- Take into consideration some of the **dyslexic difficulties** and **strengths**
- Make adjustments to **recognise** and **accommodate** the needs of dyslexic learners

The CAMEL method

When you want to make your teaching fully effective ask a **CAMEL**!

Creative – Are you appealing to the creative skills of your dyslexic learners? Ask students to find a creative way to learn or remember something.

Active – Are your learners active participants rather than passive receivers of information? What are you asking them to do?

Multi-sensory – Are your learning opportunities multi-sensory? Can you VAK them!

Effective 4 u – Do your students know what works for them? Can you raise their self-awareness about which methods work best to weaken their weaknesses and strengthen their strengths?

Learning – Are you teaching your learners how to learn?

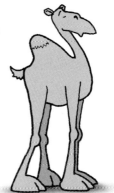

Reading

Markers
Dyslexics often have tracking problems which means they may lose their place within a line of text or within a paragraph. Using a finger or marker for keeping place within text may help. A clear or see-through bookmark is effective, as it allows the eyes to run ahead to the next words. These are available as commercial products with tinted windows. (See page 119.) You can make your own, eg from the window packaging for a packet of tights or from OHP acetates. A line ruled across the top edge with a marker pen defines the edge and it can be used lengthways to keep place.

Barrington Stoke
Barrington Stoke is a publisher specialising in fiction and resources for struggling, dyslexic, disengaged and under-confident readers. Before publication, their books are tested by the readers themselves. The books are 'dyslexia friendly'; for example they are printed on cream or off-white paper, which is more restful on the eye. They also have well-spaced text and clear and direct language structures. There are three series of books for young people aged 8-14+.   www.barringtonstoke.co.uk

Proof-reading

Dyslexic learners have difficulty **checking their work** and identifying their own mistakes. You can teach your learners to proofread more efficiently by looking for errors in only one category or by proofreading in stages using **COPS:**

Capitalisation

Omissions

Punctuation

Spelling

This may also be used as a **marking strategy** – mark for only one thing at a time or the feedback may be too overwhelming.

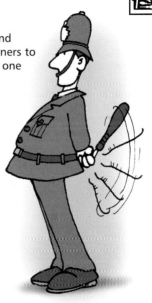

Finding information

When reading to obtain information for a project or essay, dyslexic learners often have difficulty identifying whether text is appropriate for their needs. They can use the following formula of **SQ3R** to assist them.

Survey the text. Look over the book/chapter/article. Get a feel for the subject matter. Read the 'blurb' on the back cover of a book or the outline of the article. Look at the illustrations, diagrams, graphs.

Question: Set a question, goal or aim. Sometimes you have your question set for you, sometimes you will need to ask the question such as: *'Does this article tell me about volcanoes in Italy?'*

Read the text and underline key words. Highlighter pens may be beneficial.

Recall the question. Refer back to the aim of your reading. Can your question be answered? Recall the information you have just read.

Review: Consider what has been read. Look back over the material.

Speaking and listening

Many dyslexic learners have difficulty processing spoken information.

When giving instructions:

- Keep them **short**
- Use **key pictures** and **words** to 'hook' the information on to. You can draw these pictures or symbols on the whiteboard or on a flip chart. Allow the dyslexic learner to jot down symbols or page numbers as you go through the instructions
- Be prepared to **repeat** instructions
- **Do not** expect dyslexic learners to read instructions and **copy** them from the board or screen. If it is absolutely necessary that they copy instructions out, offer a copy on paper for near rather than distant copying. It may be of little value to copy and perhaps more effective to issue, for example, a written copy of homework instructions which can be stuck or stapled directly into a diary. This will give more chance of the homework tasks being completed
- Allow dyslexic learners to **record** your instructions via a Dictaphone

Spelling magic

You can use a variety of techniques to teach dyslexics spelling. The foundation for teaching spelling must be structured and cumulative. When choosing your technique, teach your learners (and their parents) how to make the method as multi-sensory as possible.

Bear in mind that some dyslexic learners find the **look** of a word difficult to process and some find **sounds** more difficult to process, so making spelling methods multi-sensory works best.

Magical spelling
There is an NLP based technique which uses our understanding about eye movements and visualisation of words to teach spelling. Information can be found in a booklet called Magical Spelling available from www.magicalspelling.com

LSCWC

First ensure that the word is written out **correctly** and then use **LSCWC** – **L**ook, **S**ay, **C**over, **W**rite, **C**heck

LOOK: Looking does not mean a quick glance. It involves using as many senses as possible to take in the word, and make it memorable. Looking means:

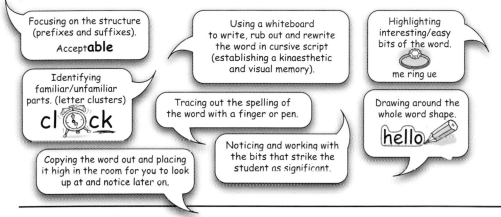

Focusing on the structure (prefixes and suffixes). Accept**able**

Using a whiteboard to write, rub out and rewrite the word in cursive script (establishing a kinaesthetic and visual memory).

Highlighting interesting/easy bits of the word. me ring ue

Identifying familiar/unfamiliar parts. (letter clusters) cl ck

Tracing out the spelling of the word with a finger or pen.

Drawing around the whole word shape. hello

Copying the word out and placing it high in the room for you to look up at and notice later on.

Noticing and working with the bits that strike the student as significant.

LSCWC

SAY means:

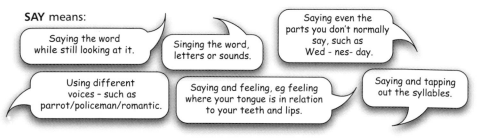

Saying the word while still looking at it.

Singing the word, letters or sounds.

Saying even the parts you don't normally say, such as Wed - nes- day.

Using different voices - such as parrot/policeman/romantic.

Saying and feeling, eg feeling where your tongue is in relation to your teeth and lips.

Saying and tapping out the syllables.

COVER the word you have learned. Try and visualise or hear it.

Keeping it covered, **WRITE** the word down. Try using:

- Different coloured pens
- Folded pieces of paper
- Big letters
- A whiteboard

Uncover the word and **CHECK** that you've reproduced it correctly. Try moving the two versions together and matching them using VAK techniques.

Using **LSCWC** in combination with multi-sensory methods like this is most effective.

Letter reversals

Dyslexic people often have trouble reproducing letters and numbers such as b and d, p and q, 5 and 2 the correct way round. This is related to visual memory and the ability to flip letters in the mind's eye. There are numerous ways to help fix the letter in the memory. Two of the most popular are:

Bed
The left hand forms the letter b and the right hand forms the letter d. This can be done by creating the 'a-ok' sign with right and left hands and bringing the thumbs together. The uprights form the bedposts.

Magic bd glasses Use the 'a- ok' method as above and bring the hands up to the eyes forming magic glasses which tell you which way round the letters go.

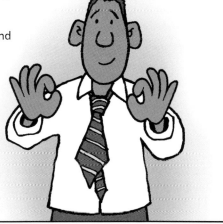

Multi-sensory mnemonics

Mnemonics are helpful for learning those odd words that dyslexics get stuck on and can also be used for a variety of information, not just for spellings.

Island = An island **is land** surrounded by water

Because = **b**ig **e**lephants **c**an't **a**lways **u**se **s**mall **e**ntrances (**because** they are so big)

Combine this method with multi-sensory techniques :

Act it out – say it – do it – feel it – think it – write it big – write it small – write it joined up – write it in the air – model it – trace it – sing it – laugh it – have fun and remember it!

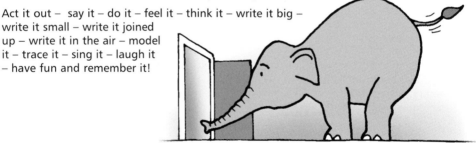

Maths

Some, but not all, dyslexic learners may have difficulty with aspects of numeracy and maths. Issues involve directional difficulties, sequencing difficulties, reading, the language of maths, maths symbols, etc.

Dyscalculia has been recognised relatively recently. It is a term used to describe a specific learning difficulty with maths but not with language. While little is currently known about the prevalence of this SpLD, research in progress is likely to shed more light on the subject in years to come.

It is important that dyslexics are taught maths in a multi-sensory way. They need to work with **concrete objects** to grasp the abstract concepts. So using Cuisenaire rods, Dienes blocks and everyday objects such as straws, pencils, sticks, etc is good practice.

9 times table

Use the finger method for the 9 times table:

1. Hold both of your hands out, palms down in front of you.

2. Tuck away the finger representing the number you are going to multiply by nine. The pictures show the sum 8 x 9. So finger 8 is tucked away.

3. Count the number of fingers to the left of the hidden finger. These represent the tens. In this case it is 7 (tens) So the answer will be seventy something.

4. Then count the fingers to the right of the hidden number. These represent the units, in this case 2.

5. So, the answer is 7 tens and 2 units which is 72.

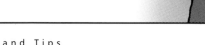

9 times table

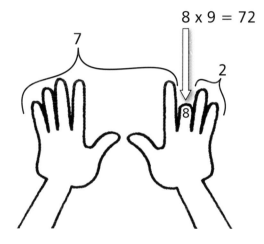

$$8 \times 9 = 72$$

7

2

8

Maths tips

- To remember the number of degrees in a triangle, announce, and get your class to announce it, like a darts commentator: *'One hundred and eighty'*

- To remember which way to plot x and y co-ordinates, teach that 'You crawl before you walk' because you always give the x co-ordinate before the y co-ordinate. The representation can also assist in recalling which is the x and y axis, as the baby is crawling across the horizontal surface and the walking man stands vertically at the side

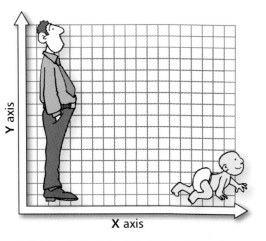

Y axis

X axis

Handwriting

Dysgraphia is the term used to refer to a specific learning difficulty with writing.

Dyslexic learners often produce handwriting that is hard to read.
Handwriting is primarily about movement not shape and when we are teaching
younger students 'letter shapes' the use of kinaesthetic techniques is vitally important.

Air writing and washing up bottles
Write the letters in the air or, using a
washing up liquid bottle filled with
water, write on the playground.
This offers safe opportunities to
get the movement right.

Hand tracing
Trace the letter shape with the
finger onto the palm of the
hand.

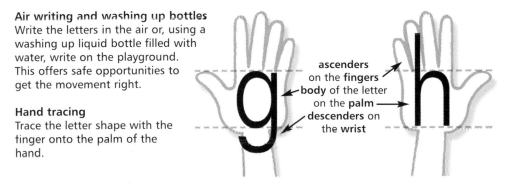

ascenders
on the **fingers**
body of the letter
on the **palm**
descenders on
the **wrist**

Improving handwriting

Be specific about what you want your student to improve

- Parallel ascenders
- Parallel descenders
- Uniform spacing between words
- Uniform spacing between letters
- Body of letters sitting on the line
- Formation of particular letters
- Joining of particular letters
- Slope of writing

Improving my writing

They can assess their own writing by using highlighter pens to focus on one of these items.
Try adjusting the grip of the writing implement with rubberised pen grips or special pens. (See Page 119.)

Modern languages

Dyslexic students face various difficulties with learning foreign languages.

Linkword Languages is a helpful resource which can be used in schools and at home. It uses an association method whereby the foreign word is linked to a visualisation of a picture of something familiar. For example:

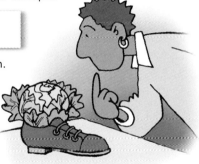

> The French word for **cabbage** is **Le Chou**.
> Imagine a **Cabbage** growing out of a **shoe**.

The CD-based resource also gives the pronunciation. Linkword is available in 12 different languages. There is a free online demonstration at www.linkwordlanguages.com

A detailed article entitled *'Modern Foreign Languages and Dyslexia: A Survivor's Guide to Languages and the National Curriculum'* can be found amongst other useful articles at www.specialeducationalneeds.com

Music

Difficult aspects of music for dyslexic learners may include the language of music, timing, laterality, sight-reading, notation, directionality, sequencing forwards and backwards, theory and recall difficulties. Try the following tips:

- Get your students to make up their own mnemonics for the treble clef lines **EGBDF**: **E**lephants **G**row **B**ig **D**angly **F**eet; the spaces **FACE**: **F**red **A**te **C**hocolate **E**ggs; and the bass clef lines **GBDFA**: **G**randpa **B**ob **D**oesn't **F**eel **A**ppreciated

- Coloured stickers and highlighters can be used in a variety of ways, eg mark where repeats start with coloured sticky arrows

- Make or buy tactile aids that represent the lengths of sounds – your student can then *feel* the length of a semibreve and compare it with a tiny semiquaver

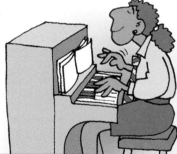

Further information about music and dyslexia is available online at www.abrsm.org where you will find an article by Sheila Oglethorpe on how to teach music to dyslexics using multi-sensory methods.

ICT as a tool

There are numerous resources available for assisting with dyslexia. It is wise to seek expert advice before buying, as different products match particular dyslexic needs. This list is not exhaustive but it includes a selection of the types of ICT help available for classroom use. (See pages 117-118 for specific products worth considering.)

Screening and assessment of dyslexia – Computerised programs are available for identifying dyslexic traits. Whilst these are suitable for screening, they cannot act as a substitute for a trained professional assessment.

Text to speech – There are two types of text reading aids:

1. Software programs for pc's which allow text to be read from computer documents.
2. Handheld devices which allow text to be read from books or paper.

Speech to text – This type of product can help with getting thoughts on to paper by dictation. There are lots of things to consider regarding speech recognition software, primarily the compatibility of your computer system, soundcard, mike etc. But also consider the user's clarity of speech and the setting in which it is going to be used.

ICT as a tool

Handheld Spellchecker – Some have thesauruses and definitions which help to identify the correct spelling of a word. Take advice about those most appropriate for particular dyslexic difficulties.

Portable word processor – A robust, cheaper alternative to a laptop.

Concept mapping program – for visual representation of thoughts, notes and planning.

PDA – for remembering names, addresses, deadlines for homework, rehearsals, etc.

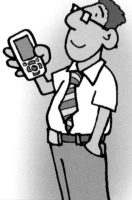

Dictaphone – for note taking, recording reminders, ideas, homework instructions.

ICT programs can be used to support literacy and numeracy skills, touch typing, word-processing skills.

The 6 Ls

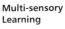

Presenting information

Teachers often ask what they can do to make information clearer for dyslexic students. There are some very straightforward methods that all teachers can easily adopt to the benefit of both dyslexic and non-dyslexic students.

When presenting (written and verbal) information to dyslexic students the following methods will help you to make your information more accessible:

1. **Legibility** – font, special fonts
2. **Layout** – space and paper
3. **Links** – link important parts of the text to key words and pictures
4. **Language** – communication and readability
5. **Large picture, little chunks** – overview and chunking down
6. **Look again, let it settle** – review and reflection

1. Legibility

Text that non-dyslexic readers might find legible is not necessarily the same thing that dyslexic learners find legible.

Ensure that the words you present on handouts, exercise books, work sheets, overhead projector or boards are dyslexia friendly.

- Handwriting needs to be **well spaced, clear, well defined**
- Typing is best read when it is a minimum **12 point** or **14 point** font size
- Underlining can make the text blur for some dyslexics
- If you need to emphasise words use **bold** or colour
- Use **lower case**, not all CAPITALS, unless a student specifically requests this. (Capitals are all the same height which means it's less easy to distinguish the letters)

1. Legibility

When you choose a font for your handouts or overheads you will probably chose one you like the look of, but some fonts are more easily legible than others.

There are **two** main forms of **typeface**:

1. **Serif** fonts are those which have little curly bits added on to the ends of the letters: like this font which is Times New Roman

2. **Sans serif** fonts are those without (sans) serif: like this font which is Arial

The font used for dyslexics should be sans serif. Sans serif fonts which come with Microsoft Word® documents are: (These are illustrated in 12pt)

Arial   Comic Sans   Trebuchet
Verdana   Tahoma

When choosing a font, it is worth making a note of how the letters 'r' and 'n' are represented. If these letters are printed too close together, in certain fonts they may look like the letter m and cause confusion for dyslexic readers.

1. Legibility

Special fonts
You can purchase some other recommended fonts:

- **Sassoon** – a typeface originally designed to make reading easier. Various types of Sassoon are available. www.clubtype.co.uk
- **APhont**™ – a typeface designed specifically for low vision readers www.aph.org

Another font designed specifically for people with dyslexia and called **Read Regular** is being developed. www.readregular.com

However, it is to some extent a personal matter: some dyslexic people report that they get used to certain fonts, such as Times New Roman, or Century School Book, despite the serif. Try experimenting with fonts and ask your students which they prefer.

2. Layout

When you plan the layout of text on a page, keep it uncluttered and limit the possibility of visual disturbance by incorporating space.

Space
- The spacing between typed lines should ideally be 1.5 spacing
- The space left at the end of lines needs to be uneven, not justified (This makes tracking across from one line to the next easier)

2. Layout

Paper
Do you ever consider the impact of your choice of paper?

- **Colour** – some dyslexics experience visual disturbance that is made worse by reading black text on a white background. A grey or off-white paper sometimes relieves this

- **Matt** paper does not create a reflection like some shiny paper. This can make reading easier

- **Not too thin!** Print from the back of double-sided sheets can show through to cause visual interference

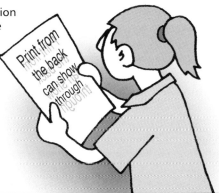

3. Links

It's easier to take information in through key words and key pictures. The brain receives information quicker from pictures than words. If you link important parts of the text to key words and pictures, you will help dyslexics to **contextualise** the information more quickly.

Key words and key pictures

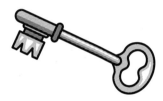

- Highlight **key words** by making them **bold**
- Put key words into summary **boxes** within the text to help your readers get an idea of what the text is about 'at a glance'
- Use **bullet points**
- Use **titles** and **sub titles**
- Use key pictures which provide a **break** for the eyes when reading (This is especially important for those experiencing visual stress)
- Insert pictures or symbols which will assist the learner in making **links** between the **text and meaning** and between the **meaning and their own experience**

4. Language

Many dyslexic learners have difficulty processing language. Take account of this in the way you communicate with your students. Use:

- **Positive language** *'Walk!'* rather than *'Stop running'*
- **Plain English** – *'Explain why'* rather than *'Explore the permutations of ...'*
- **Active language** – *'Mrs Jones decided'* rather than the passive *'It was decided'*
- **Concrete language** – Link abstracts to concrete by using similes, metaphors, stories or anecdotes
- **Open questions** – *'Are there any names you can think of ?'* rather than *'What is the name for...?'* provides the learner with the possibility of offering several answers instead of narrowing to one expected answer. You might be pleasantly surprised by creative or novel answers
- **Multi-sensory language** – Appealing to many learning preferences

Keep sentence length **short** and sentence structure **simple**.

4. Language

Readability
Check your computer-generated information for readability using tools which are provided with Microsoft ® Office Word documents:

The Flesch reading ease score
- Ideally the readability score should be between 70 – 80 out of 100
- A higher score is better than a lower score

The Flesch Kincaid grade score
- This rates your writing on an American school grade system
- A score of 7 means an 'average' 7th grader can easily understand your writing. (To convert the American grade to the English year group equivalent, add one year, eg American grade 7, plus 1 = English Year 8)

You can set up your system to automatically display the reading scores after Word has finished checking the spelling and grammar. Use the Word Help facility to find instructions on how to do this.

5. Large picture, little chunks

When presenting a lesson, new information, assembly, etc include the **large picture**. In other words, give students an **overview**; tell them what you are planning to do and why. This enables them to understand:

- What context they are learning in
- What they are going to do
- How near the beginning and end of the lesson they are

It helps them to:
- Process the learning in a holistic way
- Start to consciously or subconsciously ask predictive questions about the learning

Conveying the large picture can be done in a multi-sensory way using diagrams, Mind Maps®, acronyms or mnemonics. A good overview would convey the topic outline, the key elements and the progression.

5. Large picture, little chunks

Little chunks

If you break the learning down into steps, you create a progressive, structured approach. This enables your students:

- To make step-by-step connections between what you are teaching
- To experience learning steps which are not overwhelming
- Not to overtire from overworking a weak memory system by trying to recall large amounts of information

When you are 'chunking down' the learning:

- Relate the parts to the whole to give context
- Use **'7 plus or minus 2'** chunks of information (This is based on Miller's theory and helps with dyslexic short-term memory limitations.)
- Introduce little chunks with learning breaks

By using the **large picture, little chunks** methods you will appeal to different kinds of learning preferences and include more learners.

6. Look again, let it settle

Review

At the end of your session include a **review** of what you have just done. It only needs to take a few minutes. Present a summary of the information using:

* Memory maps®
* Pictures and symbols
* Mnemonics or acronyms (a word made up of the first letters of what you are trying to remember) eg PEE (Point, Example, Explain)
* Concert review – music playing quietly in the background as you review information
* Learning partners – pair students up to talk through a summary
* Creative methods – ask students to present summaries as newsreaders or policemen, or review it on tape like a task from 'Mission Impossible'

If you really want information to be retained in your students' long-term memory review the information regularly. Try reviewing after one hour, one day, one week, one month, and six months.

6. Look again, let it settle

Reflection

When you allow time for **reflection**, students can make meaning from the information and ask further questions when they have thought about it. This enables them to:

- Recall the recent learning
- Transfer the information to the long-term memory
- Make associations and links
- Reflect on and absorb what they have just learned
- Formulate questions which can clarify their understanding of the content

Dyslexics often find reflection time valuable because it

✓ Allows extra processing time
✓ Reinforces the learning using a different learning method
✓ Balances out the emotional response to learning by allowing a later, rational, logical response

Introduction

 What is Dyslexia?

 Dyslexia and Self-esteem

 Multi-sensory Learning

 Teaching Tools and Tips

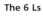 The 6 Ls

 Current Approaches ◀

 Further Resources

Current Approaches

Horses for courses

There is a wide range of approaches to help relieve the difficulties dyslexic learners experience. There may well be children in your class whose parents have introduced them to some of these. It's worth knowing about them so you can recognise what your students have been involved in and support or acknowledge their experiences.

This chapter will give you a brief overview of various approaches to dyslexia. Some are widely accepted as scientifically proven, others are not.

The fact that a method is included in this chapter does not necessarily mean that I am recommending it to you. However, I have only included those which I know dyslexics have tried and found to be useful. Different things seem to work for different people. If you or your students' parents are interested in investigating some of them further, the following tips might be useful:

- Check for **independent research** that supports the claims of the method
- Beware of **'cure all'** claims
- Talk to other **dyslexia professionals** to find out what they think of the method

Approaches based on nutrition

Some of your students may be taking nutritional supplements in order to help with their dyslexia.

Dr. Alex Richardson and Marion Ross are co-directors of a charity called FAB Research: Food And Behaviour Research. Their work explores how nutrition and diet can affect behaviour, learning and mood. One area being investigated is how **fish oils** can help dyslexics, in particular HUFA's (Highly Unsaturated Fatty Acids) Omega-3 and Omega-6 fatty acids. There is a wealth of information on the FAB website at www.fabresearch.org

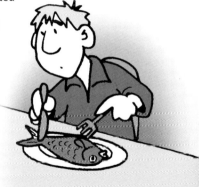

Supplements which contain these HUFA's include

- **Efalex** www.efamol.co.uk
- **eye q** www.equazen.com
- **MorEPA** www.healthyandessential.co.uk
- **OM3 Junior** www.isodisnatura.co.uk

Approaches based on vision

Some dyslexic learners experience visual disturbance, one of the many symptoms being moving or distorted text. (If you suspect any visual disturbance at all, I'd recommend your student be referred for a routine eye check first.) You may see some students with coloured overlays or coloured lenses in their glasses. These may come from various sources:

1. An Irlen centre

Helen Irlen first described Scotopic Sensitivity Syndrome or Irlen syndrome in the 1980's. It is also known as Meares-Irlen syndrome after Helen Irlen and Olive Meares. Diagnosticians use coloured overlays and lenses to reduce perception difficulties. A list of accredited Irlen diagnosticians and centres in the UK is available at www.irlenuk.com Book: *Reading By The Colours* by Helen Irlen.

2. ChromaGenTM lenses

David Harris originated the ChromaGen™ lenses from his research into the treatment of colour blindness, and Dyslexia ChromaGen™ tinted spectacles and lenses are made at Cantor and Nissel, Northants. To find out your nearest registered ChromaGen™ practitioner, telephone Cantor and Nissel on 01280 702002 or visit www.dyslexia-help.co.uk

Approaches based on vision

3. **The Intuitive Colorimeter and Overlays (Arnold Wilkins)**

   Arnold Wilkins' work is based at the Visual Perception Unit, University of Essex. There is a research & support e-group for those who suffer from 'visual stress'. www.essex.ac.uk/psychology/overlays; Tel: 01206 872 381

   The Intuitive Colorimeter is used by various local opticians to assess and supply coloured overlays and glasses. Contact Cerium Visual Technologies on 01580 765211 or visit www.ceriumvistech.co.uk for a list of optometrists using the colorimeter in your area. Cerium Visual Technologies also sells the Wilkins 'Rate of Reading Test' and the 'Colour Overlay Testing' test.

4. **The I.O.O. Institute of Optometry**

   The I.O.O. sells: Intuitive Overlays, City Coloured Overlay Screener (including a computerised version of the Wilkins Rate of Reading Test), and the City Vision Screener for Schools (a software program), all available for schools to purchase. I.O.O. 56-62 Newington Causeway, London SE1 6DS. www.ioosales.co.uk; Email: admin@ioosales.co.uk; Tel: 0207378 0330
   Book: *Reading through Colour* by Arnold Wilkins

Approaches based on vision

5. **Eye Science® UK Ltd and Tintavision (Peter Irons)**

   Eye science uses the term 'Asfedia' to describe visual difficulties accessing text and related to dyslexia. It is an acronym for Arrythmic, Saccade and Foveation during Edge Detection Iterative Arrays. Eye Science offers 'asfedic tuning' to determine which colour to use on your computer and as an overlay. Asfedic coloured note pads are also available: www.tintavision.com; Tel: 0845 130 5552

6. **Ian Jordan**

   To alleviate symptoms of 'visual dyslexia' Ian Jordan has developed:

   - The Visual Tracking Magnifier VTM (A high powered magnifying glass with a central viewing strip)

   - The Optim-Eyes Lamp (A lamp with colour and luminance adjustments)

   They are available from Edward Marcus Ltd at www.edwardmarcus.co.uk
   Ian's website is: www.visualdyslexia.com
   Books: *Visual Dyslexia: A guide for Parents and Teachers* and *Visual Dyslexia – Signs, Symptoms and Assessments* both by Ian Jordan.

Approaches based on vision

7. **The Dyslexia Research Trust**
   (Professor John Stein and Dr. Sue Fowler)
   Research and assessments for visual problems associated with dyslexia.
   Contact: Clarice Davies, University Laboratory of Physiology, Oxford, OX1 3PT
   www.dyslexic.org.uk; Email: clarice.davies@physiol.ox.ac.uk; Tel: 01865 272116

Your students may have been given, perhaps by an optometrist who is a member of the BABO, a series of exercises designed to improve their visual performance.

8. **British Association of Behavioural Optometrists (BABO)**
   Behavioural Optometry uses lenses and vision training activities to improve visual performance. Ask for your nearest accredited behavioural optometrist or see the on-line list at www.babo.co.uk; Email: info@babo.co.uk; Tel: 029 2022 8144

Approaches based on hearing/listening

Some students will have used a sound-based programme to address auditory perceptual or processing difficulties. They may have audio or computerised programmes to work through, such as:

1. **The Listening Program**® (based on the work of Dr. Alfred Tomatis)

   This is a music and sound stimulation programme designed to retrain the auditory system to improve phonological processing and many other areas of sensory organisation. It involves listening to a series of CD's, ideally twice a day for 15 minutes, for at least 8 weeks. The aim is to exercise the tiny muscles in the ear and build stronger pathways in the brain. It is said to benefit people with dyslexia as well as other learning difficulties. See:
   www.advancedbrain.co.uk and www.learning-solutions.co.uk

2. **Fast ForWord**® (Dr. Tallal and Dr. Merzenich)

   Scientific Learning Corporation at www.scilearn.com produces a series of computer-delivered programmes for students to improve speech/language skills, such as auditory memory, phonemic awareness and analysis. The UK representatives for Fast ForWord: www.innovative-therapies.com

Approaches based on hearing/listening

3. **A.R.R.O.W.** (Aural, Read, Respond, Oral, Write)

   This is a multi-sensory learning programme developed by Dr. Colin Lane. It addresses reading, spelling, speaking and listening and its key element is that the learner uses a recording of his/her own voice to facilitate learning. The student is actively involved in listening, speaking and writing. A.R.R.O.W. is based on the National Curriculum Literacy programme and delivered by CD Rom package available for schools and individuals.

   A.R.R.O.W. Centre, Crypton House, Bridgwater College, Bristol Rd, Bridgwater, Somerset, TA6 4SY www.self-voice.com; Email:drcolinlane@yahoo.co.uk; Tel: 01278 450932

4. **Software programs related to auditory/phonological processing**

   - Chatback by Xavier
   - Earobics by Cognitive Concepts
   - Lexion by Frolunda Data
   - Sounds and Rhymes by Xavier

   All available from iansyst Ltd (see page 116).

Approaches based on movement

1. **Brain Gym® and the Educational Kinesiology Foundation (Edu-K)**
   (Founders: Dr. Paul Dennison and Gail E. Dennison)

   Brain Gym® consists of 26 simple activities which can be used in a whole class or small group setting. You may know colleagues who use this approach in their classrooms, or children who practise the exercises at home.

   The official website, www.braingym.org.uk, carries a list of accredited instructors and consultants. It describes Brain Gym® as *'an educational, movement-based programme which uses simple movements to integrate the whole brain, senses and body, preparing the person with the physical skills they need to learn effectively.'*

   Educational Kinesiology UK Foundation, 12 Golders Rise, London. NW4 2HR

   Email: info@braingym.org.uk

   Book: *Brain Gym® Teachers' Edition* revised
   by Paul E. Dennison and Gail E. Dennison

Approaches based on movement

You might be aware of students practising movements at home from:

2. **The Institute for Neuro–Physiological Psychology (INPP®)**
   (Founder: Peter Blythe)
   Following a Neuro Developmental assessment the client is given an exercise
   programme which consists of a series of 'Reflex Stimulation & Inhibition'
   movements which should be carried out at home for 10 minutes a day.
   INPP offer one-day courses for teachers for implementing a special INPP schools'
   programme in a group or class activity.
   INPP Ltd, 1 Stanley Street, Chester. CH1 2LR
   www.inpp.org.uk;   Email: mail@inpp.org.uk; Tel: 01244 311414

3. **Primary Movement** (Founder: Martin McPhillips, Queen's University Belfast)
   Primary Movement is a programme involving the replication of foetal movements
   in order to help the central nervous system to mature. It is used to benefit people
   with specific learning difficulties, including dyslexia. 15 Ravenhill Road,
   Belfast BT6 8DN, Northern Ireland www.primarymovement.org;
   Email: info@primarymovement.org; Tel: 02890 222182

Approaches based on movement

Some children may have been assessed at a DDAT centre and may practise the exercises at home.

4. **DORE Achievement Centres/DDAT** (Founder: Winford Dore)
    DORE Achievement Centres offer this description of their work:
    'DORE Achievement Centres provide an exercise-based, individualised treatment programme for children and adults with specific learning difficulties such as dyslexia, dyspraxia and ADHD. After full screening and Cerebella Developmental Delay (CDD) diagnosis, the Programme involves carrying out individually prescribed exercises twice a day at home, with regular progress appointments every 6 – 8 weeks at the centre. The exercises re-train the neural pathways from the cerebellum relieving symptoms and enabling learning to become easier'.
    www.dorecentres.co.uk; Email: info@dorecentres.co.uk;   Tel:0870 880 6060

5. **Other information related to movement and learning:**
    Move it: Physical Movement and Learning by Alistair Smith. A book of practical physical movements to aid learning.
    Smart Moves: Why Learning Is Not All In Your Head by Carla Hannaford, PH D.

Approach based on perception

You may come across students who have had tuition from a Davis Practitioner.

Davis® Approach (Founder: Ron Davis)
The two components which make up Davis Dyslexia correction are:

- **Davis Orientation Counselling** ™ A technique to turn off the mental state which causes perceptual confusion with words and numbers
- **Davis Symbol Mastery** ™ A technique in which dyslexics make 3D clay models of letters, punctuation marks, words and numbers in order to make meaning for each symbol

Davis Dyslexia Correction always includes both of these components.

The Davis approach has at its heart the belief that dyslexia is a result of a mental skill or talent. To find a local practitioner, visit The Davis Dyslexia Association UK website: www.davistraining.co.uk. The international website is: www.dyslexia.com

Book: *The Gift of Dyslexia: Why Some of the Brightest People Can't Read and How They Can Learn* by Ronald D. Davis, Eldon M. Braun.

Approaches based on brain/neurology

You might find students in your class who have been involved in approaches which focus on stimulating the brain such as:

1. **BrightStar Licensing Limited**

   The BrightStar programme involves several sessions at a computer, completing a simple task with the mouse. During the process flashing lights on screen stimulate areas of the brain responsible for reading, writing and spelling. BrightStar is combined with personalised tutoring that provides a step-by-step approach to acquiring reading, writing, comprehension, and spelling skills. Some scholarships are available: www.brightstarlearning.com; Tel: 0970 3000 777

2. **Neurofeedback or EEG Biofeedback**

   In brief, Neurofeedback works by retraining the brain waves to form patterns that are most effective for learning. During the sessions, electrodes are placed on the client's scalp and in each ear. The client completes a computer game with visual and auditory feedback which can be used to help dyslexics. Information about Neurofeedback and details of the three registered UK practitioners can be found on the EEG Spectrum International website: www.eegspectrum.com

Introduction

 What is Dyslexia?

 Dyslexia and Self-esteem

 Multi-sensory Learning

 Teaching Tools and Tips

 The 6 Ls

 Current Approaches

 Further Resources

Further Resources

ICT – organisations

AbilityNet www.abilitynet.org.uk; Tel: 0800 269545
Abilitynet offers free advice and information about how technology can assist people with a variety of disabilities. Look out for the section on the website for educators. A sister site: 'my computer my way' at www.abilitynet.org.uk/myway/ explains how to customise your computer to make it more accessible to individual needs.

iansyst Ltd www.iansyst.co.uk are specialist suppliers of computers and IT solutions for people with disabilities, including those with dyslexia. Their sister site, www.dyslexic.com focuses on solutions for dyslexics. They offer free advice. Ask to speak to an educational consultant. Tel: 01223 420101

Xavier Educational Software Ltd develop and produce educational software to complement the Bangor Dyslexia Unit's teaching scheme. They are specialists in computer-based teaching aids for English language, early learning and dyslexia. School of Psychology, University of Wales, Bangor, Gwynedd, LL57 2AS Tel: 01248 382616; Email: xavier@bangor.ac.uk

ICT – products worth a look

I've indicated materials as broadly suitable for Primary (Pri) or Secondary (Sec)

Text to speech

Texthelp Read and Write is a program specifically designed for dyslexic learners allowing text to be read from any windows program. High quality speech feedback, phonetic spell-checker, word prediction dictionary and talking calculator. (Sec)

The Oxford Reading Pen is a small handheld device which scans the text and reads single words or whole lines which are then displayed on a screen and the pronunciation can be heard. This helps in recognising and pronouncing words while reading. (Sec)

Speech to text software

Dragon Dictate (Sec)

Spellcheckers

Franklin spellcheckers with UK dictionaries (Pri & Sec)

ICT – products worth a look

Organisational

Mind Manager (Sec)
Mind Genius (Sec)
Inspiration (Pri & Sec)

Touch typing

First Keys to Literacy (Pri)
Touch Type Read and Spell (Pri & Sec)
Typing Instructor Deluxe (Pri & Sec)

Numeracy and literacy

Word Shark (Pri)
Number Shark (Pri)
Nessy Learning Programme (Pri)
Star Spell (Sec)
AcceleRead AcceleWrite (Pri)
Wordbar (Top Pri and Sec)

Composition aid

Word Bar (Sec)
Visual Thesaurus by Thinkmap (Sec)

Portable word processors

Dana by AlphaSmart (Sec)
Neo by AlphaSmart (Pri)

Structured revision

Time to Revise (Pri)
Timely Reminders (Sec)

Other

Dictaphones (Pri & Sec)
Talking Books (Pri & Sec)

All the ICT resources listed here are available from iansyst.
You'll find information and advice about products at www.iansyst.co.uk

Reading rulers and pens

Inexpensive tinted 'reading rulers' are available from:

- **Eye Level Reading Rulers**: www.crossboweducation.com
- **Linetracker** www.msl-online.net Tel: 01604 505 000
- **Reading Helper**. Available from: Reading Ruler U.K. PO Box 169, Pudsey LS28 8WT
  Tel: 0113 257 7796

The Stabilo S'Move Easy pen has a moulded barrel which encourages correct and comfortable pen grip. Left and right handed versions available from www.anythingleft-handed.co.uk

The Yoropen has been designed as an ergonomic pen and provides finger support, visual space when writing, and adjustable grip. It incorporates an offset point and is suitable for both left- and right-handed writers. Available in stationers and via www.yoropen.com

Various **pen/pencil grips** are available from www.taskmasteronline.co.uk

Dyslexia/literacy teaching programmes

Alpha to Omega – The A-Z of Teaching Reading Writing and Spelling
B. Hornsby et al (Heinemann). Information from www.hornsby.co.uk

Hickey Multi-sensory Language Course – edited by J. Augur, S Briggs,
M. Combley, (Whurr Publishers) available from www.whurr.co.uk

MSL Structured Literacy Programme – devised and edited by Philippa Chudley,
published by Multi-Sensory Learning www.msl-online.net

**Toe by Toe – A Highly Structured Multi-sensory Reading Manual for Teachers and
Parents** by Keda Cowling and Harry Cowling www.toe-by-toe.co.uk

Units of Sound – information from www.dyslexia-inst.org.uk

See also:
Phonographix	www.readamerica.net
Reading Recovery	www.ioe.ac.uk
Sounds–Write	www.sounds-write.co.uk
Synthetic Phonics	www.syntheticphonics.com

Websites

Being Dyslexic	**www.beingdyslexic.co.uk**
British Dyslexia Association	**www.bda-dyslexia.org.uk**
British Dyslexics	**www.britishdyslexics.co.uk**
Dyslexia Association of Ireland	**www.dyslexia.ie**
Dyslexia Institute	**www.dyslexia-inst.org.uk**
Dyslexia International Tools & Technologies	**www.ditt-online.org**
Dyslexia Scotland	**www.dyslexiascotland.org.uk**
Helen Arkell Dyslexia Centre	**www.arkellcentre.org.uk**
Hornsby Institute	**www.hornsby.co.uk**
PATOSS	**www.patoss-dyslexia.org**
Welsh Dyslexia Project	**www.welshdyslexia.info**

The Dyslexic Teachers' Association (DTA) provides support and guidance for teachers with dyslexia http://dta42.tripod.com

If you're interested in gaining a SpLD/Dyslexia qualification, or in **training as a specialist teacher**, visit the BDA website: www.bda-dyslexia.org.uk for information.

Books

Day-to-day Dyslexia in the Classroom by Joy Pollock and Elizabeth Waller
Published by Routledge 2nd Edition 2004

Dyslexia: A Practical Guide for Teachers and Parents by Barbara Riddick,
Judith Wolfe and David Lumsdon
Published by David Fulton, 2002

How Dyslexics Learn: Grasping the Nettle by Kate Saunders and Annie White
Published by PATOSS, 2002

How to Detect and Manage Dyslexia: A Reference and Resource Manual
by Philomena Ott
Published by Heinemann Educational, 1997

Instrumental Music for Dyslexics: A Teaching Handbook by Sheila Oglethorpe
Published by Whurr, 2002

Learning to Learn Pocketbook by Tom Barwood
Published by Teachers' Pocketbooks, 2005

Maths for the Dyslexic: A Practical Guide by Anne Henderson
Published by David Fulton, 1998

Books and specialist booksellers

Overcoming Dyslexia by Dr. Beve Hornsby
Published by Vermillion, 1996

Removing Dyslexia as a Barrier to Achievement by Neil MacKay
Published by SEN Marketing, 2005

Teaching Handwriting - A Guide for Teachers and Parents by Jean Alston and Jane Taylor
Published by Qed Publications, 2000

What to Do When You Can't Learn Your Times Tables by Steve Chinn
Published by Egon Publishers, 1997

Better Books – specialist books on ADHD, Aspergers, autism, dyslexia, dyscalculia, dyspraxia.
www.dyslexiabooks.co.uk Email: sales@betterbooks.com Tel: 01384 253276

SEN Marketing – dyslexia and special needs bookshop
www.sen.uk.com   Email: info@sen.uk.com   Tel: 01924 871697

A final note

If you have a student in your class who is, or who may be, dyslexic and you'd like further advice on how to move forward with an assessment or in making appropriate provision, there are various routes to take:

- Speak with the **SENCO** (Special Educational Needs Coordinator) at your school
- Obtain a copy of the **Dyslexia Friendly Schools pack** www.bda-dyslexia.org.uk
- Seek advice about the procedures for special provision, statementing etc from
- **IPSEA: Independent Panel for Special Education Advice** www.ipsea.org.uk
- **Parent Partnership** www.parentpartnership.org.uk

Providing effective education for dyslexic students is best done through a partnership between professionals and parents. Specific extra support/ provision is available for some dyslexics in schools, depending on the degree to which they are affected. This may involve a statement of special needs, extra small group work and/or special arrangements in exams. Whether dyslexic learners have a 'statement' or not, they can all be assisted by the methods outlined in this book.

Acknowledgements and references

- A definition of dyslexia used with kind permission of Dr Lindsay Peer (page 17)
- Self-esteem definition based on the work of Dr Nathaniel Branden (page 37) used with kind permission
- *One Hundred and Eighty* used with kind permission of Peter Mansfield (page 80)
- 'Handtracing' idea used with kind permission of Melvyn Ramsden of www.realspelling.com (page 81)
- Tactile Aids representing the lengths of sounds in teaching music used with kind permission of Sheila Oglethorpe (page 84)
- Thanks to iansyst for their advice regarding ICT

I am also grateful to:

- Fran and Norman Brown, Vanessa Charter and Geoff Dowell for helping me establish my roots and wings
- Brian, Ruth and Andrew for their support and encouragement

About the author

Julie Bennett BA Hons, PCGE, Dip SpLD

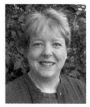

Julie is an independent consultant, working under the business name of Unlocking Potential. She started her working life as a primary school teacher and has 20 years' experience in the field of education. She has specialised in the field of dyslexia and learning. Julie works with learners of all ages and their teachers and trainers. She has a passion for unlocking potential and empowering learners.

For further information about her training she can be contacted at:
Julie@key4u.co.uk   01234 781 698   www.key4u.co.uk

Julie Bennet

Order Form

Your details

Name _____

Position _____

School _____

Address _____

_____

_____

Telephone _____

Fax _____

E-mail _____

VAT No. (EC only) _____

Your Order Ref _____

Please send me:

		No. copies
Dyslexia	Pocketbook	
_____	Pocketbook	
_____	Pocketbook	
_____	Pocketbook	
_____	Pocketbook	

Order by Post

Teachers'
Pocketbooks

Laurel House, Station Approach
Alresford, Hants. SO24 9JH UK

Order by Phone, Fax or Internet

Telephone: +44 (0)1962 735573
Facsimile: +44 (0)1962 733637
E-mail: sales@teacherspocketbooks.co.uk
Web: www.teacherspocketbooks.co.uk

Pocketbooks